# LAB VALUES, FLUIDS, ELECTROLYTES, & ACID BASE NCLEX-RN REVIEW:

100 Practice Questions with Detailed Rationales Explaining Correct & Incorrect Answer Choices

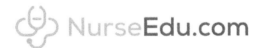

**Disclaimer:**

Although the author and publisher have made every effort to ensure that the information in this book was correct at press time, the author and publisher do not assume and hereby disclaim any liability to any party for any loss, damage, or disruption caused by errors or omissions, whether such errors or omissions result from negligence, accident, or any other cause.

This book is not intended as a substitute for the medical advice of physicians. The reader should regularly consult a physician in matters relating to their health and particularly with respect to any symptoms that may require diagnosis or medical attention.

All rights reserved. No part of this publication may be reproduced, distributed, or transmitted in any form or by any means, including photocopying, recording, or other electronic or mechanical methods, without the prior written permission of the publisher, except in the case of brief quotations embodied in critical reviews and certain other noncommercial uses permitted by copyright law.

NCLEX®, NCLEX®-RN, and NCLEX®-PN are registered trademarks of the National Council of State Boards of Nursing, Inc. They hold no affiliation with this product.

Some images within this book are either royalty-free images, used under license from their respective copyright holders, or images that are in the public domain.

ISBN: 978-1-952914-12-6

# FREE BONUS

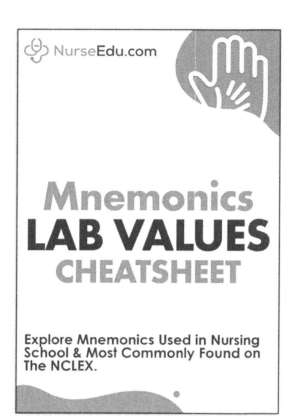

**FREE Download – Just Visit:**

**NurseEdu.com/bonus**

# TABLE OF CONTENTS

# CHAPTER 1:

## NCLEX-RN – ADULT LAB VALUES - 50 QUESTIONS

1.  A 10-year-old female patient is admitted to the emergency room in sickle cell crisis. Which of the following lab results should be reported to the healthcare provider by the nurse?

    A. Creatinine 2.8 mg/dL

    B. Hematocrit 31%

    C. Sodium 148 mEq/L

    D. White blood cells 13,000/mm$^3$

    **Rationale:**

    Correct answer: A.

Sickle cell disease is the abnormal formation of red blood cells into a sickle shape, which makes it difficult to absorb and transport oxygen through the bloodstream. This leads to breathing difficulty, pain, and end organ damage. Kidney damage is indicated by elevated creatinine levels which often occurs in patients with sickle cell disease.

B is incorrect because low hematocrit is not unusual with sickle cell disease. Normal hematocrit for a child (up to age 12) is 35-45%.

C is incorrect because the sodium is slightly elevated, possibly indicating dehydration, which is problematic for a sickle cell patient (Normal sodium is 135-145 mEq/L). Hydration status should be assessed, but kidney damage is the main concern.

D is incorrect because the normal white blood cell count for a child (up to age 12) is 5,000-13,000/mm$^3$. Sickle cell patients *are* at risk for infection, so WBCs should be monitored, and if they rise above 13,000/mm$^3$, the health care provider should be notified.

2.  The nurse on the medical-surgical unit is caring for a patient who suddenly becomes confused and starts mumbling. Upon reviewing the lab results, the nurse

finds the platelet count is 8,000/mm³. Which action should the nurse take first?

A. Call the Rapid Response Team
B. Obtain a set of vital signs
C. Institute bleeding precautions
D. Place the patient on bedrest

**Rationale:**

Correct answer: A.

Normal platelet count is 150,000-450,000/mm³. The patient is at risk for spontaneous bleeding with such a low platelet count. The patient's neurologic change could be a result of bleeding in the brain or elsewhere in the body (resulting in decreased oxygenation to the brain), so the Rapid Response Team (RRT) should be notified for assistance. Other signs of bleeding may include petechiae, bruising or visible bleeding.

B is incorrect because vital signs are important, but not the priority. The nurse has enough information (neurological decline, low platelets) to call for help. Postponing the call to the RRT will delay safe patient care. Vital signs can be taken after the RRT is called.

C is incorrect because instituting bleeding precautions is important, but not the priority over calling for immediate help at the bedside.

D is incorrect because placing the patient on bedrest is important for safety, but not the priority.

3. The nurse reviews labs in the cardiac clinic. Which of the following indicates the greatest risk for atherosclerosis?

   A. Patient takes niacin daily, triglyceride level 250 mg/dl
   B. Patient takes garlic daily and LDL is 79 mg/dl
   C. Patient admitted with angina and lab results show elevated creatine-kinase-MB
   D. Alanine aminotransferase (ALT) level 60

**Rationale:**

Correct answer: A.

Elevated triglycerides indicate increased risk for atherosclerosis, the thickening and hardening of the arteries. Normal triglycerides are 100-160 mg/dl. Niacin is taken to help reduce triglycerides, LDL, total cholesterol, and increase HDL. Elevated triglycerides indicate the niacin is not effective.

B is incorrect because LDL of 79 mg/dl is good. Garlic is often taken to reduce the risk for atherosclerosis. Because garlic can cause the blood to thin, the patient should be monitored for bleeding and thrombocytopenia.

C is incorrect because creatine kinase-MB supports a diagnosis of myocardial infarction and can help determine severity and when damage occurred, but does not indicate risk for atherosclerosis.

D is incorrect because ALT does not determine risk for atherosclerosis. Normal ALT is generally 7-56 units/L. Elevated ALT suggests liver injury, damage, or dysfunction.

4. Which lab result for a 56-year-old male patient with atherosclerosis should concern the nurse?

    A. Total cholesterol 125 mg/dL
    B. High density lipoprotein cholesterol 46 mg/dL
    C. Low density lipoprotein cholesterol 64 mg/dL
    D. Triglycerides 200 mg/dL

**Rationale:**

Correct answer: D.

Atherosclerosis refers to the buildup of fatty deposits, hardening, and stenosis (narrowing) of arteries. It is caused by increased levels of cholesterol, low density lipoprotein, and triglycerides. Total cholesterol is calculated by adding HDL, LDL, and 20% triglyceride level. In order to prevent cardiovascular effects, total cholesterol should be less than 200 mg/dL, LDL less than 130 mg/dL, and HDL greater than 40 mg/dL. Triglycerides of male patients should be less than 160 mg/dL.

A is incorrect because cholesterol 125 mg/dL is considered normal for an adult male.

B is incorrect because HDL 46 mg/dL is considered normal for an adult male.

C is incorrect because LDL 64 mg/dL is considered normal for an adult male.

5. The nurse is monitoring a patient after a total thyroidectomy. The nurse notes HR 122 bpm, BP 170/120 mm/Hg, temperature 102.5°F (39.2°C), and respiratory rate 24/minute. Which of the following interventions is the priority?

   A. Administer morphine 4mg IV

   B. Administer levothyroxine

   C. Encourage intake of cold PO fluids

   D. Administer propylthiouracil

**Rationale:**

Correct answer: D.

Tachycardia, elevated blood pressure, pyrexia, and tachypnea indicate a thyroid storm (also known as thyrotoxic crisis). This can occur after a thyroidectomy procedure, which can cause an excessive release of thyroid hormones as the gland is being surgically manipulated. This is an acute, life-threatening, hypermetabolic state. Sodium iodide, propylthiouracil (PTU) and beta-blockers are used to treat thyroid crisis.

A is incorrect because morphine is used to treat postoperative pain. The patient may be in pain, but treatment of other physical symptoms is the greater priority.

B is incorrect because levothyroxine is a thyroid replacement medication, which will worsen thyroid storm. Thyroid replacement medications will not be used until the storm has been treated and the patient's blood thyroid hormone level is reduced.

C is incorrect because during a thyroid storm, the patient may need to be kept NPO. Assessment of airway and swallowing ability must be performed before allowing PO fluids. The safest way to reduce the temperature is to use a cooling mattress or blanket.

6. The nurse cares for a patient after a lung biopsy has been performed. Which of the following actions is most important?

    A. Check vital signs every 8 hours for 24 hours and report respiratory distress to the healthcare provider

    B. Change the clean dressing once daily and assess for drainage

    C. Assess the urine for ketones

    D. Ensure chest X-ray has been taken

**Rationale:**

Correct answer: D.

A lung biopsy is performed to remove lung tissue for culture or cytology. After the procedure, a chest X-ray is routinely taken to assess for potential pneumothorax.

A is incorrect because vitals should be monitored every 4 hours for 24 hours after a lung biopsy.

B is incorrect because a sterile dressing is applied after a lung biopsy.

C is incorrect because ketones in the urine are unrelated to a lung biopsy procedure.

7. The nurse is assessing the arterial blood gas values for a patient with type I diabetes who was admitted with a blood glucose level of 750 mg/dl. Which of the following results indicates diabetic ketoacidosis?

A. pH 7.37, $HCO_3^-$ 23 mEq/L, $PCO_2$ 39 mm Hg, $PO_2$ 97 mm Hg

B. pH 7.26, $HCO_3^-$ 17 mEq/L, $PCO_2$ 27 mm Hg, $PO_2$ 99 mm Hg

C. pH 7.49, $HCO_3^-$ 29 mEq/L, $PCO_2$ 39 mm Hg, $PO_2$ 98 mm Hg

D. pH 7.31, $HCO_3^-$ 23 mEq/L, $PCO_2$ 59 mm Hg, $PO_2$ 79 mm Hg

**Rationale:**

Correct answer: B

In DKA, the ABG would reflect metabolic acidosis with a pH level below 7.35 and a low bicarbonate level. A decreased carbon dioxide level is due to compensatory respiratory alkalosis (the lungs blow off extra $CO_2$ to rid the body of acids.)

A is incorrect because the values represent a normal ABG.

C is incorrect because the results demonstrate metabolic alkalosis (high pH with high bicarbonate level), which is not an indication of DKA.

D is incorrect because the results demonstrate respiratory acidosis (low pH, high $CO_2$) with hypoxia ($PO_2$ 79), which is not indicative of metabolic acidosis seen with DKA.

8. The nurse is preparing to administer a glucose tolerance test to a patient with a suspected pancreatic tumor. Which of the following statements is appropriate for the nurse to make?

   A. "Increased physical activity will be encouraged after you drink the glucose liquid."
   B. "Regular insulin will be administered via IV, and then blood samples will be drawn at certain intervals."
   C. "Limiting carbohydrate intake over the next three days will help with the accuracy of this test."
   D. "After 2 hours, the normal blood glucose level should be about 140 mg/dl."

   **Rationale:**

   Correct answer: D.

   A glucose tolerance test measures the body's ability to secrete insulin in response to hyperglycemia. After the fasting level is drawn, the patient is instructed to drink a liquid glucose solution, after which blood glucose levels are drawn at 2 hours (and sometimes at subsequent time intervals.) A normal result at 2 hours is 140 mg/dl. A patient with a pancreatic tumor will often have an impaired glucose tolerance test.

A is incorrect because increased physical activity may affect the results of the test. The patient will remain seated or resting for the duration of the test.

B is incorrect because a glucose tolerance test does not routinely involve the administration of IV insulin. Only if the patient becomes severely hyperglycemic will insulin be administered.

C is incorrect because carbohydrates should not be limited in the days prior to the glucose tolerance test. The patient is instructed to fast for 8-12 hours before the test (NPO except for water). The test is commonly done in the morning, as glucose tolerance can decrease in the afternoon.

9. The nurse in the intensive care unit (ICU) is monitoring a patient who is scheduled for a dose of furosemide IV and digoxin. The current potassium level is 2.6 mEq/L. What is the most appropriate action by the nurse?

   A. Administer the digoxin as ordered, and then re-check the potassium level

B. Obtain a serum calcium level

C. Supplement with potassium before administering the furosemide and digoxin

D. Consult with dietary to increase potassium in the diet

**Rationale:**

Correct answer: C.

When the serum potassium level falls below 3.5 mEq/L, the patient may begin to experience muscle weakness, nausea, vomiting, paresthesia, and dysrhythmias. Potassium should be supplemented before giving the next dose of furosemide, which can further cause potassium levels to decrease.

A is incorrect because hypokalemia increases the risk for digoxin toxicity. The potassium level should be restored to normal before administering the digoxin.

B is incorrect because assessing calcium is unrelated to hypokalemia.

D is incorrect because replacing the potassium IV is more appropriate than making dietary changes. Administration of supplemental potassium will have a more immediate effect on the hypokalemia than waiting for the next meal to arrive.

10. A patient on the medical unit who has diabetes mellitus is on an intense insulin regimen. The nurse reviews the following lab results: fasting blood sugar 75 mg/dL, postprandial blood sugar 140 mg/dL, hemoglobin $A_{1c}$ 5.4%. How does the nurse interpret these results?

    A. Increased risk of ketoacidosis
    B. Good blood sugar control
    C. Increased risk of hyperglycemia
    D. Insulin resistance

**Rationale:**

Correct answer: B.

Normal fasting blood glucose is 70-100 mg/dl. A normal post-prandial blood glucose is 90-140 mg/dl. Normal hemoglobin $A_{1c}$ is 4-6%. The results are good for an intense insulin regimen, as all levels are within the defined normal ranges.

A is incorrect because the levels are good and the patient is not at increased risk of ketoacidosis.

C is incorrect because the levels are good and the patient is not at increased risk of hyperglycemia.

D is incorrect because the levels are good and the patient is not experiencing insulin resistance.

11. A female patient with gastric cancer will have a total gastrectomy performed. Which of the following preoperative lab results would the nurse expect to see before the procedure?

   A. Albumin 6.6 g/dL
   B. Hematocrit 55%
   C. Hemoglobin 10 g/dL
   D. Increased International Normalized Ratio (INR)

**Rationale:**

Correct answer: C.

Normal hemoglobin for women is 12-16 g/dL. Gastric cancer commonly causes low hemoglobin.

A is incorrect because normal albumin is 3.5-5.5 g/dL and decreased albumin is expected with gastric cancer.

B is incorrect because a normal female hematocrit is 35-47%. High hematocrit is indicative of dehydration, which is not expected prior to a gastrectomy. Gastric cancer commonly causes low hematocrit.

D is incorrect because INR is a measure of bleeding time and is routinely checked for patients taking warfarin. Increased INR is not expected before a gastrectomy procedure. If this level is elevated, the patient is at risk for bleeding and the surgeon should be notified immediately.

12. A patient admitted to the emergency room has a serum creatinine level of 2.4 mg/dL and blood urea nitrogen (BUN) of 26 mL/dL. What is the first question the nurse should ask when documenting patient history?

   A. "Have you taken aspirin, naproxen, or ibuprofen recently?"
   B. "Does anyone in your family have renal failure?"
   C. "Have you been following a low protein diet?"
   D. "Has anyone in your family had a kidney transplant recently?"

**Rationale:**

Correct answer: A.

Normal creatinine for an adult is 0.7-1.4 mg/dL, and normal BUN is 10-20 mg/dL. Both of these lab tests, when elevated, can indicate impaired renal function. Nonsteroidal anti-inflammatory drugs (aspirin, naproxen, and ibuprofen) are nephrotoxic and can elevate creatinine and BUN. The nurse should determine if the patient has taken any of these medications recently.

B is incorrect because family history of renal failure is not pertinent to this situation.

C is incorrect because a high protein diet can elevate BUN.

D is incorrect because a family history of kidney transplants is not pertinent to this situation.

13. A patient in the intensive care unit (ICU) has a potassium level 6.4 mmol/L, creatinine 2.2 mg/dL, and a urine output of 325 mL/day. Which action should the nurse take first?

   A. Initiate cardiac monitoring
   B. Teach the patient about limiting high-potassium foods
   C. Monitor intake and output
   D. Redraw blood specimen for retesting

**Rationale:**

Correct answer: A.

A normal serum potassium level is 3.5-5.0 mmol/L (3.5-5.0 mEq/L). The patient's potassium is very high. Hyperkalemia can contribute to dysrhythmias, so the patient needs to be put on the cardiac monitor. Normal creatinine for an adult is 0.7-1.4 mg/dL. When creatinine is elevated, this can indicate impaired renal function.

B is incorrect because teaching the patient about a low-potassium diet is not a priority.

C is incorrect because this patient's urine output is low (normal urine output is 30-60 mL/hr, up to 1500 mL/day), but cardiac monitoring is a greater priority.

D is incorrect because no information is given to suggest that the blood sample needs to be redrawn. The safest action is to immediately begin monitoring for cardiac changes.

14. The nurse is planning to care for a patient receiving total parenteral nutrition (TPN). Which of the following lab studies would the nurse plan to monitor most frequently?

   A. White cell count and differential count

B. Hemoglobin and hematocrit

C. Liver function studies

D. Blood glucose and urine specific gravity

**Rationale:**

Correct answer: D.

Blood glucose should be checked every 6 hours when a patient is receiving TPN. The patient is at increased risk for hyperglycemia. Urine specific gravity should also be checked 2-4 times daily for osmotic diuresis, which increases the risk for dehydration.

A is incorrect because white cell count and differential count should be checked weekly to monitor for sepsis. These labs may be checked more frequently if the patient exhibits signs of infection.

B is incorrect because hemoglobin and hematocrit should be checked daily until a constant volume of TPN is infused.

C is incorrect because liver function studies should be checked weekly for a patient receiving TPN. AST, ALT, and serum alkaline phosphates may be elevated due to excessive glycogen deposits in the liver.

15. The nurse evaluates care for a patient who has been treated for adrenal insufficiency. Which of the following changes indicates that the patient is not responding favorably to treatment?

   A. Urinary output has decreased.

   B. Blood pressure has increased.

   C. The patient has lost weight.

   D. The patient's sodium level has increased.

**Rationale:**

Correct answer: C.

In adrenal insufficiency, a lack of adrenocorticotropic hormones leads to fluid depletion, increased urine output, drop in blood pressure, dehydration, weight loss, sodium loss, and hyperkalemia.

A is incorrect because a decrease in urinary output is a sign the patient is responding favorably to hormone treatment.

B is incorrect because hypotension is a symptom of adrenal insufficiency. Volume restoration is a goal of therapy, and thus the nurse would monitor blood pressure closely. Increase in blood pressure is a sign of responding favorably to treatment.

D is incorrect because increase in sodium level indicates a positive response to treatment.

16. A patient has arterial blood gas results as follows: pH 7.26, $PaO_2$ 54 mm Hg, $PaCO_2$ 66 mm Hg, and $HCO_3$- 23 mEq/L. Which of the following interventions should the nurse implement?

    A. Decrease the patient's oxygen flow rate
    B. Administer 50 mL of sodium bicarbonate intravenously
    C. Encourage the patient to hyperventilate
    D. Assess if the patient has experienced any recent diarrhea

**Rationale:**

Correct answer: C.

This patient is experiencing severe respiratory acidosis. The normal bicarbonate level indicates that this is not metabolic. This patient has inadequate gas exchange given the elevated $PaCO_2$. Encouraging hyperventilation will help open the alveoli and get rid of the excess $CO_2$.

A is incorrect because the patient is hypoxic and the oxygen flow rate should be increased.

B is incorrect because the patient's bicarbonate level is normal and the nurse's priority is to address respiratory needs first.

D is incorrect because diarrhea leads to metabolic acidosis and is not related to respiratory acidosis with hypoxia.

17. The nurse is caring for a patient with chronic renal failure. Which of the following results from this morning's lab draw is most concerning to the nurse?

   A. Serum potassium 5.0 mEq/L
   B. Serum sodium 134 mEq/L
   C. Serum calcium 7.5 mg/dL
   D. Serum phosphorus 2.3 mEq/dl

   **Rationale:**

   Correct answer: C.

Normal serum calcium is 8.5-10.5 mg/dl. In chronic renal failure, hypocalcemia occurs as a result of the body trying to compensate for increased serum phosphorus. (Calcium and phosphorus have a reciprocal relationship; as one rises, the other decreases.) Hypocalcemia can lead to uremic bone disease, also known as osteodystrophy.

A is incorrect because the potassium levels are within normal range. In chronic renal failure, hyperkalemia occurs due to decreased excretion of potassium from the kidneys and metabolic acidosis.

B is incorrect because, although this is not a normal sodium level, it is only slightly low. High sodium with chronic renal failure is more concerning to the nurse. Hypernatremia results from malfunction of the renin-angiotensin-aldosterone system.

D is incorrect because a normal serum phosphorus level is 2.5-4.5 mEq/dl. Chronic renal failure often causes an increased phosphorus level.

18. A patient newly diagnosed with type 1 diabetes calls the clinic nurse to report a rise in blood glucose at 3 AM over

the previous 3 nights. Which of the following instructions are appropriate for the nurse to give?

A. Change the time of the evening intermediate-acting insulin to earlier in the evening
B. Change the evening intermediate-acting insulin from dinnertime to bedtime
C. Discontinue the evening snack
D. Increase calorie intake at the bedtime snack

**Rationale:**

Correct answer: B.

If blood glucose is relatively normal until about 3 AM when levels begin to rise, this is likely Dawn Phenomenon. The evening intermediate-acting insulin should be given later.

A is incorrect because giving the intermediate-acting insulin earlier will not treat Dawn Phenomenon.

C is incorrect because discontinuing the evening snack will not prevent the Dawn Phenomenon from occurring and can lead to bedtime hypoglycemia.

D is incorrect because increase in bedtime snack is indicated for the Somogyi Effect (hypoglycemia between 2-3 AM and then a subsequent increase in blood glucose due to counterregulatory hormone action).

19. The nurse is caring for a patient who has recently been admitted for acute alcohol withdrawal. Which of the following findings indicates the patient has severe alcoholic cirrhosis?

    A. Albumin 3.3 g/dl
    B. Total serum bilirubin 0.9 mg/dl
    C. Absence of ascites
    D. Prothrombin Time (PT) 18 seconds

**Rationale:**

Correct answer: D.

Severe alcoholic cirrhosis is characterized by poor nutritional state, albumin less than 3.0 g/dl, bilirubin greater than 3.0 mg/dl, poorly controlled ascites, and prolonged prothrombin time (PT). Normal PT is 9.5-12 seconds.

A is incorrect because normal serum albumin is 3.5-5.5 g/dl. Severe alcoholic cirrhosis is characterized by albumin less than 3.0 g/dl.

B is incorrect because normal total serum bilirubin is 0-0.9 mg/dl. Severe alcoholic cirrhosis is often characterized by increased bilirubin level, due to the liver's inability to conjugate and excrete bilirubin.

C is incorrect because ascites worsens as liver function deteriorates with severe cirrhosis.

20. The nurse is caring for a patient with cardiac disease. When discussing lab results, the patient asks "What is the significance of my high BUN level?" What is the appropriate response by the nurse?

    A. "I will call the healthcare provider to come discuss your lab results with you."
    B. "The bronchodilators that you take can cause an increased BUN level."
    C. "The elevated BUN can be an indication that your kidneys are not receiving enough blood flow."
    D. "Your diuretic medication should help decrease your BUN level."

**Rationale:**

Correct answer: C.

Normal BUN is 10-20 mg/dl. In patients with cardiac disease, an elevated BUN can indicate reduced renal perfusion (from decreased cardiac output) or intravascular fluid volume deficit (from diuretic therapy.)

A is incorrect because the nurse should discuss the concerns with the patient. Calling the healthcare provider to the room is only appropriate after the nurse determines that the patient's questions cannot be answered by the nursing staff.

B is incorrect because bronchodilators do not cause an increase in BUN. Side effects of bronchodilators include headache, nervousness, tremors, and palpitations.

D is incorrect because diuretics can be the cause of dehydration, leading to an increased BUN. Diuretic medications will not likely correct an increased BUN level.

21. A patient is experiencing extreme anxiety with hyperventilation, blood pressure 170/95 mm Hg, pulse

122 bpm, and respiratory rate 25/minute. The patient has the following arterial blood gas results: pH 7.30, $PaO_2$ 94, $PaCO_2$ 31, and $HCO_3$- 26 mEq/L. Which intervention should the nurse implement?

A. Assess the patient's history of anxiety attacks
B. Have the patient breathe fast and hard, with forced expiration
C. Encourage the patient to calm down
D. Teach the patient to breathe into a paper bag

**Rationale:**

Correct answer: D.

Anxiety and hyperventilation can lead to respiratory alkalosis, as seen in the ABG, so the nurse should focus on correcting the breathing. Breathing into a closed system, such as a paper bag, will help the patient accumulate $CO_2$ and correct the alkalosis.

A is incorrect because assessing a history of anxiety is not the priority. The nurse should focus on correcting the here-and-now problem, which is current anxiety and respiratory alkalosis.

B is incorrect because forceful expiration will further cause $CO_2$ levels to decrease and worsen the patient's alkalosis.

C is incorrect because it does not address the alkalosis immediately. It may be unrealistic to expect a very anxious patient to simply "calm down" when instructed. The nurse should implement measures that directly address the breathing.

22. The nurse is caring for a patient experiencing right-upper quadrant pain, jaundice, and confusion. Acetaminophen poisoning is suspected. Which of the following interventions is appropriate?

    A. Limit fluids

    B. Check kidney function studies

    C. Prepare the patient for a cardiac stress test

    D. Draw blood to check for white blood cell count

**Rationale:**

Correct answer: B.

A patient being treated for acetaminophen poisoning needs adequate hydration and N-acetylcysteine-specific antidote. Liver function studies (AST, ALT) and kidney function tests (creatinine, BUN) are also required.

A is incorrect because increased fluids are indicated for acetaminophen poisoning to maintain hydration.

C is incorrect because a cardiac stress test is not indicated for a patient with suspected acetaminophen poisoning.

D is incorrect because WBC count is not a priority for acetaminophen overdose.

23. A patient is receiving intravenous heparin for pulmonary embolism (PE). The most recent partial thromboplastin time (PTT) result was 110 seconds. What does the nurse anticipate as the next action?

    A. Decrease the heparin infusion rate
    B. Increase the heparin infusion rate
    C. No change to the heparin infusion rate
    D. Stop the heparin infusion and administer warfarin

**Rationale:**

Correct answer: A.

When on a heparin infusion, the therapeutic PTT should be 1.5 to 2.5 times normal. Normal PTT is 20 to 39 seconds, so this patient's PTT result is too high. The heparin infusion should be decreased to prevent excessive bleeding.

B is incorrect because the PTT is too high and increasing the heparin rate will lengthen the PTT.

C is incorrect because the PTT is too high and the heparin infusion needs to be decreased.

D is incorrect because warfarin is not indicated.

24. The nurse is assessing a patient for Trousseau's sign. Which of the following will indicate a positive Trousseau's sign?

A. Tap cranial nerve 7 and cranial nerve 5 and check for facial grimace
B. Place a blood pressure cuff on the arm and check for carpopedal spasms when cuff is inflated
C. Check deep tendon reflexes by tapping the knee
D. Monitor the patient for nausea when cold water is used to irrigate ear canal

**Rationale:**

Correct answer: B.

Trousseau's sign indicates hypocalcemia and is elicited by placing a blood pressure cuff on the upper arm and inflating to 20 mm Hg above the patient's normal systolic blood pressure. Carpopedal spasms with cuff inflation indicates a positive result (hypocalcemia).

A is incorrect because this is a part of assessing Chvostek's sign.

C is incorrect because deep tendon reflexes are not part of Trousseau's sign.

D is incorrect because cold water ear canal irrigation is not part of Trousseau's sign. With cold water ear irrigation, the nurse will expect to see nystagmus in the eyes while the cold water is instilled into the ear canal. Absence of nystagmus indicates damage to the nerves of the inner ear or brain.

25. A patient with a history of diabetes is admitted to the emergency department with dilated pupils. Which action by the nurse indicates an understanding of the presenting symptom?

   A. Check Hgb $A_{1C}$

   B. Begin IV of normal saline

C. Apply oxygen via mask at 3 liters per minute

D. Give the patient 240 mL of apple juice

**Rationale:**

Correct answer: D.

Hypoglycemia is indicated by an altered level of consciousness, dilated pupils, and cool and clammy skin. Juice will elevate blood glucose levels. If the patient is too drowsy to take PO fluids, IV glucose can be administered.

A is incorrect because checking Hgb $A_{1C}$ will not correct hypoglycemia. Hgb $A_{1C}$ is checked to determine blood glucose control over the past three months.

B is incorrect because IV normal saline will not correct hypoglycemia. Administration of normal saline is not contraindicated, but raising the patient's blood glucose is the greatest priority.

C is incorrect because oxygen will not correct hypoglycemia.

26. A screen test for detection of human immunodeficiency virus (HIV) reveals a positive ELISA (enzyme-linked immunosorbent assay) test. After the healthcare

provider explains the results to the patient, the nurse will prepare the patient for which of the additional tests?

A. Radioimmunoprecipitation assay (RIPA) test

B. HSV-2 (herpes simplex virus 2) antibody detection test

C. Total lymphocyte count

D. Indirect immunofluorescence assay (IFA)

**Rationale:**

Correct answer: D.

After a positive ELISA test, an HIV diagnosis can be confirmed by Indirect immunofluorescence assay (IFA) or a Western blot test.

A is incorrect because (similarly to the ELISA test) RIPA detects HIV protein, but does not confirm a diagnosis.

B is incorrect because HSV-2 is not the cause of HIV. HSV-2 antibodies indicate genital herpes, not HIV.

C is incorrect because lymphocytes are used to detect progression of the illness, not confirm diagnosis. Lymphopenia, thrombocytopenia, and anemia are expected as HIV progresses.

27. A patient taking digitalis has laboratory tests drawn. Which of the following results does the nurse report to the healthcare provider?

   A. Sodium 138 mEq/L

   B. Chloride 98 mEq/L

   C. Potassium 3.0 mEq/L

   D. Digoxin level 0.8 ng/mL

**Rationale:**

Correct answer: C.

A normal serum potassium level is 3.5-5.0 mEq/L, and hypokalemia can increase the risk for digitalis toxicity. The healthcare provider should be notified, and the nurse should anticipate administration of a potassium supplement before the next dose of digitalis is given. Digitalis is a cardiac glycoside medication, which strengthens the force of myocardial contraction. It also slows the heart rate by stimulating the vagus nerve and blocking the AV node.

A is incorrect because normal sodium is 135-145 mEq/L.

B is incorrect because normal chloride is 96-108 mEq/L.

D is incorrect because a therapeutic digoxin level is 0.5-2.0 ng/mL. Blood levels in excess of 2.0 ng/mL indicate toxicity.

28. A female 19-year-old patient who sustained head trauma during a motor vehicle accident is admitted to the emergency department. The nurse notes 2,000 mL of dilute urinary output within 3 hours of admission. Which of the following findings is most important for the nurse to communicate to the healthcare provider?

    A. Erythrocytes 6.0 x 10$^{12}$ L
    B. Urine specific gravity 1.005
    C. Blood urea nitrogen 8 mg/dl
    D. Serum creatinine 0.5 mg/dl

    **Rationale:**

    Correct answer: B.

    Diabetes insipidus (DI) is a dangerous complication of head trauma, caused by a decreased production or release of the antidiuretic hormone, which results in polyuria with low specific gravity (less than 1.010). This needs to be communicated to the healthcare provider so that vasopressin can be ordered and administered to help reduce fluid loss and correct dehydration.

A is incorrect because normal red blood cell (RBC) count for a woman is 4.2-5.4 x $10^{12}$/L. A high erythrocyte count can indicate dehydration, which can occur with DI, but the specific gravity is more important to communicate with the healthcare provider.

C is incorrect because normal blood urea nitrogen is 10-20 mg/dl. Low BUN may indicate fluid volume overload, which is unrelated to head trauma or diabetes insipidus.

D is incorrect because normal serum creatinine is 0.7-1.4 mg/dl. Low creatinine is not a complication of head trauma or an indication of DI.

29. A patient is admitted to the medical-surgical unit after a thyroidectomy procedure. The patient's post-operative calcium level was 7.2 mg/dL, and although the patient was treated with calcium gluconate, seizure activity has started. Which of the following actions is most appropriate for the nurse to take?

   A.  Increase milk products in the diet

B. Increase the light in the room to allow for close observation

C. Recheck serum calcium level

D. Administer phenobarbital

**Rationale:**

Correct answer: D.

After a thyroidectomy, the parathyroid glands may have been injured. Hypoparathyroidism is manifested by decreased calcium levels and can cause seizures. After calcium gluconate is administered, and in the instance that neuromuscular irritability and seizure activity are still present, sedatives such as phenobarbital are to be used. Normal calcium is 8.4-10.2 mg/dL.

A is incorrect because, although milk products are high in calcium, dietary concerns are not the greatest priority during the post-operative hypoparathyroid management.

B is incorrect because light and stimulation in the patient's room should be limited when calcium levels are low and seizure activity is present.

C is incorrect because immediate intervention is necessary ahead of rechecking labs. No information is present to indicate a need for rechecking calcium.

30. A patient diagnosed with congestive heart failure (CHF) has a scheduled dose of furosemide. Which lab value should the nurse report to the healthcare provider before administering the furosemide?

    A. Potassium 5.0 mEq/L
    B. Sodium 133 mEq/L
    C. Ionized calcium 4.2 mg/dl
    D. Potassium 3.3 mEq/L

**Rationale:**

Correct answer: D.
Normal potassium is 3.5-5.0 mEq/L, and furosemide is a loop diuretic that causes potassium excretion. Hypokalemia can be dangerous as it can cause fatal heart arrhythmias, especially for patients with CHF.

A is incorrect because the potassium level is normal.

B is incorrect because the sodium level is slightly low, but not a reason to withhold the furosemide. Normal sodium is 135-145 mEq/L.

C is incorrect because the normal ionized calcium level is 4.5-5.1 mg/L. Slightly decreased ionized calcium is not a reason to call the healthcare provider before administering furosemide.

31. A patient's laboratory results are reviewed by the nurse. Which results should indicate to the nurse that the patient may have atherosclerosis? (Select all that apply)

   A. Total cholesterol 290 mg/dL
   B. High density lipoprotein cholesterol 52 mg/dL
   C. Triglycerides 205 mg/dL
   D. Serum albumin 5 g/dL
   E. Low density lipoprotein cholesterol 170 mg/dL

**Rationale:**

Correct answer: A, C, E.

Lipid panels are used when screening for cardiovascular risk. Lipids and cholesterol form plaque buildups within the cardiac vessels, leading to stenosis and blockage. This patient's total cholesterol, triglycerides, and LDL are all elevated, indicating an increased risk for cardiovascular disease.

B is incorrect because HDL 52 mg/dL is normal.

D is incorrect because albumin is not related to triglycerides. Normal serum albumin is 3.5-5.5 g/dl.

32. Which of the following assessments indicate improvement in a patient with left-sided heart failure? (Select all that apply)

   A. Hematocrit: 32.8%
   B. Serum sodium: 152 mEq/L
   C. Absence of protein in the urine
   D. Microalbuminuria
   E. Lung sounds clear and equal bilaterally
   F. Moderate ascites

**Rationale:**

Correct answer: C, E

Proteinuria is a sign of heart failure, and thus, lack of protein in the urine is a sign of improvement. Clear lung sounds indicate lack of fluid in the lungs, which is a good assessment in a heart failure patient.

A is incorrect because the hematocrit is low, which indicates dilutional anemia and is consistent with heart failure.

B is incorrect because dilutional hyponatremia with fluid overload is seen with heart failure. Hypernatremia is not a sign of improvement.

D is incorrect because microalbuminuria indicates renal filtration is decreased, which is a sign of continuing heart failure.

F is incorrect because, although ascites is often seen in right heart failure, it is not an improvement in a patient with left heart failure.

33. The nurse is caring for a patient in the emergency room who may have hyperaldosteronism. The patient complains of fatigue and headache. Which of the following does the nurse expect to find? (Select all that apply)

    A. Sodium 133 mEq/L
    B. Sodium 155 mEq/L
    C. Magnesium 3.1 mEq/L
    D. Potassium 2.6 mEq/L
    E. Decreased urine output
    F. Blood pH 7.48

    **Rationale:**

    Correct answer: B, D, F.

    Hyperaldosteronism results in hypernatremia, hypokalemia, and metabolic alkalosis.

    A is incorrect because hyponatremia is associated with adrenal insufficiency.

    C is incorrect because hypomagnesemia is associated with hyperaldosteronism.

E is incorrect because polyuria is associated with hyperaldosteronism.

34. The nurse is caring for a patient admitted for hyperparathyroidism. The morning lab results show a calcium level of 11.2 mg/dl. Which of the following does the nurse expect to observe? (Select all that apply)

    A. Fatigue
    B. Neuromuscular excitability
    C. Diarrhea
    D. Hypotension
    E. Cardiac dysrhythmias

**Rationale:**

Correct answer: A, E.

Hyperparathyroidism causes hypercalcemia, which has the following clinical manifestations: fatigue, muscle weakness, nausea, vomiting, constipation, hypertension, and cardiac dysrhythmias.

B is incorrect because muscle weakness will be present.

C is incorrect because constipation is more likely than diarrhea.

D is incorrect because hyperparathyroidism and hypercalcemia will cause an increase in blood pressure.

35. The nurse cares for a 65-year-old male patient with liver disease. The lab results show increased international normalized ratio (INR), increased serum ammonia, and prolonged prothrombin time (PT). Based on these lab values, the nurse knows the patient is at risk for which of the following? (Select all that apply)

    A. HIV infection
    B. Deep vein thrombosis
    C. Neuromuscular excitability
    D. Risk for injury
    E. Confusion
    F. Hemorrhage

    **Rationale:**

    Correct answer: D, E, F.

    Increased PT and INR indicate clotting disorders (decreased ability of the blood to clot) and could lead to hemorrhage. The liver normally converts ammonia into urea, which is then eliminated in urine. Increased ammonia in the blood will cause fatigue, muscle weakness, loss of appetite, nausea, vomiting, diarrhea, and pain in the back, sides or abdomen. Increased confusion puts the patient at risk for injury.

A is incorrect because the lab values do not pose an increased risk for HIV infection.

B is incorrect because the patient is at risk for bleeding, not clotting.

C is incorrect because increased ammonia will cause muscle weakness, not excitability.

36. The nurse is caring for a patient admitted for glomerulonephritis. The patient is taking PO fluids and has an IV of 00.9% NS running at 50 mL/hr. When reviewing the patient's 24-hour creatinine clearance results, the nurse finds that the glomerular filtration rate (GFR) is 115 mL/minute. What is the appropriate action that the nurse should take?

   A. Notify the healthcare provider
   B. Document the GFR
   C. Increase the patient's IV fluid rate
   D. Discontinue the IV fluids

**Rationale:**

Correct answer: B.

GFR is a measurement of kidney filtering function. Normal GFR is 100-120 mL/min, much of which the kidney tubules reabsorb. This patient's GFR at 115 mL/min is within the normal expectation, so documenting the results is appropriate.

A is incorrect because the healthcare provider does not need to be notified of normal lab results.

C is incorrect because a normal GFR does not warrant an increase in IV fluids. A patient taking PO fluids with an additional 50 mL/hr of NS is most likely receiving enough fluids to meet the daily fluid needs. An increase in fluid rate could lead to fluid volume retention.

D is incorrect because a normal GFR is not an indication for discontinuing IV fluids. It is not within the scope of practice to discontinue fluids unless a medical emergency is present.

37. A patient with peptic ulcer disease has been taking omeprazole for 11 years. The patient comes to the clinic complaining of muscle weakness, and lab results show a

magnesium level of 0.9 mg/dl. Which of the following does the nurse expect to observe in this patient? (Select all that apply)

A. Depressed deep tendon reflexes

B. Hypotension

C. Tremors

D. Dizziness and impaired breathing

E. Nystagmus

F. Increased neuromuscular activity

**Rationale:**

Correct answer: C, E, F.

Omeprazole is a proton-pump inhibitor used to treat GI ulcers. Long-term use of proton-pump inhibitor medication can lead to magnesium deficiency. Hypomagnesemia can cause neuromuscular irritability, tremors, tetany, seizures, dysrhythmias, depression, confusion, and dysphagia.

A is incorrect because decreased deep tendon reflexes would be seen with hypermagnesemia, not hypomagnesemia.

B is incorrect because hypotension would be expected with hypermagnesemia, not hypomagnesemia.

D is incorrect because dizziness and impaired respiratory function are seen with high magnesium levels, not hypomagnesemia.

38. The nurse is caring for a patient with severe sepsis. The patient has a triple lumen central venous pressure (CVP) catheter in place. The CVP catheter can be used for which of the following? (Select all that apply)
    A. Antibiotic administration
    B. To obtain an arterial blood gas sample
    C. Intravenous fluid infusions
    D. Measurement of pulmonary artery (PA) pressure
    E. To obtain blood cultures

**Rationale:**

Correct answer: A, C, E.

A triple lumen CVP catheter can be used to measure CVP (pressure in the right atrium of the heart) as a way of monitoring fluid status for a patient who is hemodynamically unstable. The nurse can use the CVP catheter to infuse fluids and medications, to obtain venous blood samples for lab testing, and to measuring CVP.

B is incorrect because the CVP catheter is placed in a vein, not an artery. Thus, obtaining an arterial blood sample is not possible through this catheter.

D is incorrect because PA pressure must be measured by using a PA catheter placed in the pulmonary artery, not by using a CVP catheter.

39. The nurse is reviewing lab results for a patient who had a lumbar puncture performed earlier in the day. Which of the following cerebrospinal fluid (CSF) results are abnormal? (Select all that apply)

    A. Pink-colored CSF
    B. Red blood cells present in the CSF
    C. CSF protein 60 mg/dl
    D. CSF glucose 60 mg/dl
    E. CSF lactic acid < 24 mg/dl

**Rationale:**

Correct answer: A, B, C.

Cerebrospinal fluid (CSF) is typically a clear and colorless fluid with a specific gravity of 1.007. Normally, CSF has a minimum number of white blood cells present, and no red blood cells. The normal protein level in a lumbar sample of CSF is 15-45 mg/dl. If the protein level is greater than 45 mg/dl, this can be characteristic of tubercular meningitis.

D is incorrect because the normal level of glucose in CSF is 50-75 mg/dl. Increased glucose in the CSF can indicate diabetes mellitus or can be seen in diabetic coma. Decreased glucose in the CSF can indicate meningitis or insulin shock.

E is incorrect because this is a normal level of lactic acid in CSF. Increased lactic acid (>24 mg/dl) in CSF can indicate bacterial meningitis or hydrocephalus.

40. A patient is receiving a continuous intravenous infusion of heparin sodium to treat deep vein thrombosis. The patient's activated partial thromboplastin time (aPTT) is 37 seconds. Based on this result, which of the following interventions does the nurse anticipate performing? (Select all that apply)

    A. Maintain the rate of the heparin infusion.
    B. Decrease the rate of the heparin infusion.
    C. Increase the rate of the heparin infusion.

D. Discontinue the heparin infusion.

E. Administer a heparin bolus.

**Rationale:**

Correct answer: C, E.

Normal aPTT is 20-39 seconds. For deep vein thrombosis treatment, therapeutic range is aPTT level between 1.5 and 2.5 times normal, so the aPTT should not be less than 30 or greater than 97 seconds. The current aPTT of 37 seconds is too low, so the nurse should anticipate increasing the rate of the heparin infusion and administering a bolus.

A is incorrect because the aPTT is too low and maintaining the current heparin infusion rate will not increase the aPTT to a therapeutic level.

B is incorrect because the aPTT is too low and decreasing the rate of the heparin infusion will be ineffective in treating the DVT and thus will be detrimental to the patient.

D is incorrect because the aPTT is too low and the patient needs a continuous heparin infusion to treat the DVT.

41. A patient admitted with suspected hypoparathyroidism has labs drawn. Which of the following results correlate with hypoparathyroidism? (Select all that apply)

    A. Serum potassium 3.2 mEq/L
    B. Serum calcium 0.8 mEq/L
    C. Serum phosphorus 5.7 mg/dL
    D. Serum magnesium 1.7 mg/dL
    E. Serum chloride 88 mEq/L

**Rationale:**

Correct answer: B, C.

Hypoparathyroidism causes decreased calcium absorption and elevated phosphate levels. Normal calcium is 8.4-10.2 mg/dL, and normal phosphorus is 3.0-4.5 mg/dL.

A is incorrect because the potassium level is low, and hypokalemia is unrelated to hypoparathyroidism.

D is incorrect because the magnesium level is normal and unrelated to hypoparathyroidism.

E is incorrect because the chloride level is low, and decreased chloride is unrelated to hypoparathyroidism.

42. A patient is admitted to the emergency room with chest pain and shortness of breath. Which of the following lab results indicate that the patient is experiencing myocardial infarction? (Select all that apply)

   A. Myoglobin 98 mcg/L
   B. Troponin T 0.09 ng/mL
   C. Troponin I 2.0 ng/mL
   D. Creatine kinase (CK-MB) 180 units/L
   E. Myoglobin 4 mcg/L

   **Rationale:**

   Correct answer: A, C, D.

   Myocardial infarction is diagnosed by the presence of elevated myoglobin, troponin I, and CK-MB, which are all elevated in this patient. Normal myoglobin is 5-70 mcg/L, normal troponin I is <0.035 ng/mL, and normal CK-MB is 55-170 units/L.

   B is incorrect because the troponin T level is normal.

   E is incorrect because the myoglobin level is normal.

43. The nurse on the telemetry unit is reviewing lab results for a patient receiving digoxin and notes the digoxin level

is 2.5 ng/mL. The nurse plans to do which of the following? (Select all that apply)

A. Administer the next scheduled dose of digoxin

B. Notify the healthcare provider

C. Check the patient's pulse rate

D. Administer an additional loading dose of digoxin per protocol

E. Hold the next digoxin dose

F. Assess the patient's pupils in response to light

**Rationale:**

Correct answer: B, C, E.

Normal therapeutic range for digoxin is 0.5-2 ng/mL, so 2.5 indicates toxicity. The nurse should notify the healthcare provider and anticipate holding the next dose, as well as checking the patient's pulse rate for bradycardia. Digoxin is a cardiac glycoside which works by strengthening the force of myocardial contraction and slows the heartrate. The heartrate can drop to a dangerously low rate in the case of digoxin toxicity.

A is incorrect because the digoxin level is high so the next dose should be withheld.

D is incorrect because the digoxin level is high so an additional dose is unnecessary.

F is incorrect because assessing pupil response is not a necessary nursing action for a patient with digoxin toxicity.

44. A patient in the emergency department has a sodium level of 119 mEq/L. The patient has an IV of 0.45% NaCl running at 75 mL/hr. After checking all other lab values, which of the following does the nurse perform? (Select all that apply)

    A. Change the IV fluid to 0.9% NaCl
    B. Notify the healthcare provider
    C. Teach the patient about high-sodium meal options
    D. Check deep tendon reflexes for hyperreflexia
    E. Check for Trousseau's sign

**Rationale:**

Correct answer: A, B, C.

The normal serum sodium level is 135-145 mEq/L, so the patient has hyponatremia. It is an appropriate nursing action to change the IV fluid to one that contains a greater concentration of sodium. The healthcare provider should be notified and the nurse should teach the patient about high-sodium meal options. Foods high in dietary sodium include processed foods, lunchmeats, dairy products, canned items, and carbonated beverages.

D is incorrect because deep tendon reflexes would be hypoactive with hyponatremia.

E is incorrect because Trousseau's sign is unrelated to hyponatremia. Trousseau's sign is elicited by placing a blood pressure cuff on the upper arm and inflating to 20 mm Hg above the patient's normal systolic blood pressure. Carpopedal spasms with cuff inflation indicates hypocalcemia.

45. An adult patient is taking rosiglitazone for diabetes. Which lab result(s) should be reported to the healthcare provider? (Select all that apply)

   A. Blood glucose 110 mg/dL
   B. Creatinine 3.0 mg/dL
   C. Blood urea nitrogen level 30 mg/dL
   D. White blood cell count 8,000/mm$^3$
   E. Amylase 25 units/L

**Rationale:**

Correct answer: B, C.

Rosiglitazone is a thiazolidinedione oral antidiabetic medication. This drug can lead to renal and liver failure. Normal creatinine is 0.7-1.4 mg/dL and normal blood urea nitrogen is 10-20 mg/dL, so both are elevated in this patient.

A is incorrect because the blood glucose is within the normal range, 70-110 mg/dl.

D is incorrect because the white blood cell count is within the normal range for an adult, 5,000-10,000/mm³.

E is incorrect because the amylase level is within the normal range, 0-137 U/L. Increased amylase levels are typically seen with pancreatitis.

46. An adult male patient is admitted to the emergency department following a motor vehicle accident in which he sustained a laceration to the lower right leg and extensive hemorrhage. Which lab result(s) would the nurse expect to find? (Select all that apply)

A.  Hemoglobin 14.2 g/dL

B.  Hematocrit 34%

C.  White blood cell 6,000/mm³

D.  Platelets 510,000/mm³

E.  Red blood cell 3.9 million/mm³

## Rationale:

Correct answer: B, E.

Trauma with massive bleeding will lead to decreased hemoglobin, decreased hematocrit, and decreased red blood cell counts. In males, normal hemoglobin is 13-18 g/dl, hematocrit is 42-52%, and red blood cells are 4.6-6.2 million/mm³.

A is incorrect because the hemoglobin is within normal expectations for an adult male. The patient who has experienced severe hemorrhaging would have decreased hemoglobin.

C is incorrect because the white blood cell count is within the normal range for an adult, 5,000-10,000/mm³. The patient, who has experienced trauma, would have an elevated WBC count due to the inflammatory response. (Even in the absence of infection, WBCs will migrate to an area that has been damaged in attempts to repair the tissue.)

D is incorrect because the platelet count is elevated, which is not expected after trauma and hemorrhage. Normal platelets are 150,000-450,000/mm³.

47. The nurse in the clinic is assessing lab values for a patient with hypercholesterolemia. Which of the following results does the nurse expect to find? (Select all that apply)

    A. Total cholesterol 190 mg/dL
    B. Low density lipoprotein (LDL) 150 mg/dL
    C. High density lipoprotein (HDL) 35 mg/dL
    D. Triglycerides 200 mg/dL
    E. Albumin 3.7 g/dL

**Rationale:**

Correct answer: B, C, D.

Hypercholesterolemia is elevated cholesterol, which is evaluated using total cholesterol, LDL, HDL, and triglycerides. The normal values are: total cholesterol <200 mg/dL, LDL <70 mg/dL, HDL >60 mg/dL, and triglycerides <150 mg/dL.

A is incorrect because the total cholesterol is normal.

E is incorrect because albumin is unrelated to hypercholesterolemia.

48. A patient is admitted to outpatient surgery for a traditional liver biopsy. Which of the following lab tests does the nurse anticipate performing to assess coagulation? (Select all that apply)

    A. Partial thromboplastin time (PTT)
    B. Prothrombin time (PT)
    C. Platelet count
    D. Hemoglobin
    E. Complete blood count

**Rationale:**

Correct answer: A, B, C.

Coagulation studies include PTT, PT, and platelet count.

D is incorrect because hemoglobin does not assess coagulability of the blood. Hemoglobin measures the oxygen-carrying capacity of the blood.

E is incorrect because complete blood count does not assess coagulation.

49. The nurse is evaluating a patient's response to hemodialysis. Which lab results will indicate that dialysis was effective? (Select all that apply)

A. Serum potassium change from 5.4 to 4.6 mEq/L

B. Creatinine change from 1.9 to 0.8 mg/dL

C. Hemoglobin change from 10-12 g/dL

D. White blood cell change from 9,000 to 19,000/mm$^3$

E. Blood urea nitrogen change from 80 to 45 mg/dL

**Rationale:**

Correct answer: A, B, E.

Hemodialysis is primarily performed to clear nitrogenous waste products from the blood. Lab results that indicate effectiveness of dialysis include decreased potassium, decreased creatinine, and decreased blood urea nitrogen.

C is incorrect because hemoglobin does not indicate hemodialysis effectiveness.

D is incorrect because white blood cells do not indicate hemodialysis effectiveness. An elevated WBC level after dialysis indicates potential infection.

50. The nurse in the hemodialysis center is caring for patients. The nurse understands that which of the following lab results are indications for dialysis? (Select all that apply)

A. Blood urea nitrogen 18 mg/dL

B. Potassium 5.2 mEq/L

C. Creatinine clearance 70 mL/min

D. Metabolic acidosis

E. Creatinine 4.0 mg/dL

**Rationale:**

Correct answer: B, C, D, E.

Hemodialysis is primarily performed to clear nitrogenous waste products. Indications for dialysis include increased potassium, decreased creatinine clearance, metabolic acidosis, and increased creatinine. Normal potassium is 3.5-5.5 mEq/L. Normal creatinine clearance is 97-137 ml/min (for males). Normal serum creatinine for adults is 0.7-1.4 mg/dl.

A is incorrect because the blood urea nitrogen is normal (10-20 mg/dl). Dialysis is indicated when BUN level rises abnormally high and cannot be decreased by other nursing and medical interventions.

# CHAPTER 2:

# NCLEX-RN – FLUIDS, ELECTROLYTES, & ACID-BASE IMBALANCE - 50 QUESTIONS

1.  The nurse in the emergency room is caring for a 38-year-old male who has had nausea and vomiting for 3 days. The nurse knows this patient is most likely experiencing:

    A.  Respiratory acidosis

    B.  Respiratory alkalosis

    C.  Metabolic acidosis

    D.  Metabolic alkalosis

    **Rationale:**

    Correct answer: D.

Metabolic alkalosis occurs when hydrogen ions (acids) are lost and bicarbonate ($HCO_3-$) concentration (base) increases. This causes an increase in the pH balance of the blood to greater than 7.45. Vomiting (loss of GI acids) commonly results in dehydration and metabolic alkalosis, especially when prolonged.

A is incorrect because respiratory acidosis does not occur from nausea and vomiting. Respiratory acidosis results from accumulation of $CO_2$, a respiratory acid.

B is incorrect because respiratory alkalosis occurs from a loss of $CO_2$, not from nausea and vomiting.

C is incorrect because metabolic acidosis results when kidneys fail to properly excrete non-respiratory acids, not from nausea and vomiting.

2. A patient with chronic renal failure is admitted due to a decreased level of consciousness and Kussmaul respirations. Lab tests are drawn and the patient has an acid-base imbalance. Which statement is most appropriate for the nurse to make to the patient?

A. "You may be suffering from respiratory acidosis, in which your lungs are holding on to too much carbon dioxide."

B. "Respiratory alkalosis is likely in this case because your kidneys aren't excreting acids."

C. "Your body is currently prone to metabolic acidosis, and your breathing is an attempt to get rid of excess acids."

D. "Metabolic alkalosis is common in renal patients, but we will be sure to give you the best care possible."

**Rationale:**

Correct answer: C.

Metabolic acidosis occurs when hydrogen ions increase and bicarbonate ($HCO_3-$) concentration decreases. This causes the pH balance of the blood to fall to less than 7.35. Chronic renal failure commonly causes metabolic acidosis due to the inability of the kidneys to make bicarbonate and properly excrete acids from the circulatory system. Kussmaul respirations compensate for acidosis and are slow, deep respirations that decrease levels of carbon dioxide, an acid.

A is incorrect because chronic renal failure causes metabolic acidosis, not respiratory acidosis.

B is incorrect because respiratory alkalosis is not an effect of chronic renal failure. Respiratory alkalosis occurs when the lungs excrete too much $CO_2$, an acid, leading to an increase in pH and resulting in an acidotic state.

D is incorrect because chronic renal failure does not cause commonly cause metabolic alkalosis. (The second part of the statement is therapeutic, but it is more important for the nurse to give factual information than to offer comfort and hope.)

3. A surgical patient in the recovery room is difficult to wake. The patient's SpO2 is 89%, the blood pressure measured in the left arm is 86/60 mm Hg, and the pulse is 114 bpm. Which of the following most likely explains what the patient is experiencing?

   A. Respiratory acidosis
   B. Respiratory alkalosis

C. Metabolic acidosis

D. Metabolic alkalosis

**Rationale:**

Correct answer: A.

Respiratory acidosis occurs when the post-operative patient does not breathe sufficiently, allowing carbon dioxide (acid) to accumulate in the blood. When the carbon dioxide level increases, this leads to a decrease in the pH balance of the blood to less than 7.35. As pH decreases, this causes vasodilation, which decreases blood pressure. Tachycardia is a compensatory mechanism.

B is incorrect because respiratory alkalosis occurs when a patient is breathing heavily and expelling too much $CO_2$.

C is incorrect because metabolic acidosis does not fit the symptom of this post-operative patient.

D is incorrect because the patient's imbalance is respiratory, not metabolic.

4. A patient admitted to the emergency room is experiencing anxiety, pallor, tachypnea, and tingling in the hands. The nurse knows this patient is most likely experiencing which of the following?

   A. Respiratory acidosis
   B. Respiratory alkalosis
   C. Metabolic acidosis
   D. Metabolic alkalosis

**Rationale:**

Correct answer: B.

Respiratory alkalosis occurs when a patient experiences tachypnea, which decreases carbon dioxide levels (breathing at a rapid rate expels too much $CO_2$, an acid) and therefore increases the pH balance of the blood to greater than 7.45. Respiratory alkalosis causes tingling of the hands and fingers.

A is incorrect because the symptoms do not fit respiratory acidosis. (Respiratory acidosis results from a buildup of $CO_2$ in the blood.)

C is incorrect because metabolic acidosis generally results from altered kidney function and is not primarily related to respirations.

D is incorrect because metabolic alkalosis is more likely due to prolonged vomiting, in which the body loses HCl from the stomach.

5. The nurse is assessing the arterial blood gas values for a patient with diabetes mellitus. Which of the following results would the nurse correlate with potential ketoacidosis?

   A. pH 7.37, $HCO_3^-$ 23 mEq/L, $PCO_2$ 39 mm Hg, $PO_2$ 97 mm Hg

   B. pH 7.26, $HCO_3^-$ 17 mEq/L, $PCO_2$ 27 mm Hg, $PO_2$ 99 mm Hg

   C. pH 7.49, $HCO_3^-$ 29 mEq/L, $PCO_2$ 39 mm Hg, $PO_2$ 98 mm Hg

   D. pH 7.31, $HCO_3^-$ 23 mEq/L, $PCO_2$ 59 mm Hg, $PO_2$ 89 mm Hg

**Rationale:**

Correct answer: B.

Blood pH levels decrease below normal as the lungs lose their ability to correct acidosis. A patient with diabetic ketoacidosis would have blood gas values with primarily metabolic acidosis, decreased bicarbonate level, and compensatory respiratory alkalosis as seen with decreased carbon dioxide level.

A is incorrect because the results are normal.

C is incorrect because the results demonstrate metabolic alkalosis (the bicarbonate is elevated, causing the higher pH).

D is incorrect because the results demonstrate respiratory acidosis (the low pH is caused by the elevated $CO_2$).

6. A patient with an acid-base imbalance has the following arterial blood gas results: pH 7.33, $PaO_2$ 86 mm Hg, $PaCO_2$ 38 mm Hg, and $HCO_3$- 19 mEq/L. Which nursing assessment should be performed first?

    A. Cardiac rate and rhythm

    B. Skin and mucous membranes

    C. Musculoskeletal strength

    D. Level of orientation

**Rationale:**

Correct answer: A.

This patient is experiencing moderate acidosis related to low bicarbonate (and exhibited by low pH). Early signs include cardiovascular changes, such as tachycardia and increased cardiac output. When acidosis worsens, heart rate decreases and changes on the patient's cardiac monitor will be noticed.

B is incorrect because skin and mucous membrane assessment is not priority but may become more of a concern if acidosis worsens.

C is incorrect because musculoskeletal strength changes will not occur with mild acidosis, but should be monitored.

D is incorrect because CNS changes do not occur with mild acidosis, but should be monitored.

7. The nurse is caring for a patient admitted for acid-base imbalance with the following arterial blood gas results: pH 7.32, $PaO_2$ 85 mm Hg, $PaCO_2$ 34 mm Hg, and $HCO_3$- 16 mEq/L. What is the next action the nurse should take?

A. Assess patient's rate, rhythm, and depth of respiration

B. Measure the patient's pulse and blood pressure

C. Document the findings and continue to monitor

D.  Notify the healthcare provider as soon as possible

**Rationale:**

Correct answer: A.

The low pH indicates an acidotic state, and the low bicarbonate indicates this is metabolic in nature. The slightly decreased $CO_2$ (acid) levels suggest that the respiratory system is compensating by decreasing acid retained by the lungs. Muscle weakness can occur with acidosis, which can lead to respiratory insufficiency, as progressive skeletal muscle weakness is directly associated with increasing acidosis. Thus, assessing the patient's breathing is the priority.

B is incorrect because assessing pulse and blood pressure is not a greater priority than assessing the respiratory system. The nurse's main concern is determining if the patient has enough muscular strength to breathe effectively.

C is incorrect because findings should be documented, but intervention is necessary. Direct patient care is a greater priority than documentation.

D is incorrect because the nurse needs to assess the patient for more information before notifying the healthcare provider.

8. A patient has the following arterial blood gas results: pH 7.16, $PaO_2$ 54 mm Hg, $PaCO_2$ 66 mmHg, and $HCO_3$- 23 mEq/L. Which of the following clinical situations should the nurse correlate with these values?

   A. Diabetic ketoacidosis in a person with emphysema
   B. Bronchial obstruction related to aspiration of a hot dog
   C. Anxiety-induced hyperventilation in an adolescent
   D. Diarrhea for 36 hours in an older, frail woman

**Rationale:**

Correct answer: B.

This patient is experiencing severe respiratory acidosis with hypoxia, indicated by a very low pH, low oxygen, and a high $CO_2$ level. The bicarbonate level is normal, so the nurse can rule out a metabolic cause. The elevated $PaCO_2$ can result from an inadequate gas exchange related to respiratory obstruction.

A is incorrect because DKA causes metabolic acidosis; the values represented in the scenario above indicate respiratory acidosis, not metabolic.

C is incorrect because hyperventilation leads to decreased $PaCO_2$ level and respiratory alkalosis.

D is incorrect because diarrhea leads to metabolic acidosis due to the loss of bases from the GI tract. Remember, pancreatic juice enters the small intestine to help neutralize acidic stomach contents, so a patient excreting a lot of diarrhea is losing alkalotic bicarbonate ions, leading to metabolic acidosis.

9. A patient who experienced a 90 second tonic-clonic seizure has the following arterial blood gas values: pH 6.90, $PaO_2$ 48 mm Hg, $PaCO_2$ 62 mm Hg, and $HCO_3$- 24 mEq/L. What is the first action the nurse should take?

   A. Apply oxygen by mask or nasal cannula
   B. Apply a paper bag over the patient's nose and mouth
   C. Administer 50 mL of sodium bicarbonate intravenously

D. Administer 50 mL of 20% glucose and 20 units of regular insulin

**Rationale:**

Correct answer: A.

This patient has experienced acute respiratory acidosis from excess skeletal muscle contraction with no gas exchange. The patient is also severely hypoxic. Applying oxygen is the fastest way for the nurse to restore acid-base imbalance after a seizure.
B is incorrect because a paper bag over the mouth would worsen acidosis. (A paper bag is used to treat respiratory alkalosis in patients who are hyperventilating and losing $CO_2$.)

C is incorrect because the patient does not require treatment with sodium bicarbonate as the bicarbonate level in the ABG sample is normal.

D is incorrect because glucose and insulin are initiated to correct a high potassium level, which is unknown for this patient.

10. A patient on the medical unit has the following arterial blood gas values: pH 7.49, $PaO_2$ 97 mm Hg, $PaCO_2$ 27 mm Hg, and $HCO_3$- 22 mEq/L. Which of the following

conditions should the nurse correlate with these arterial blood gas results?

A.  Diarrhea and vomiting for 36 hours

B.  Anxiety-induced hyperventilation

C.  Chronic obstructive pulmonary disease (COPD)

D.  Diabetic ketoacidosis and emphysema

**Rationale:**

Correct answer: B.

This patient's high pH indicates alkalosis, while the low $CO_2$ is likely from hyperventilation. Thus, this is respiratory alkalosis (the bicarbonate and $PaO_2$ are normal).

A is incorrect because diarrhea leads to metabolic acidosis due to the loss of bicarbonate ions from the GI tract. Vomiting can lead to alkalosis due to the loss of acids from gastric juice in stomach contents. Neither vomiting nor diarrhea generally cause respiratory acid-base imbalances.

C is incorrect because COPD leads to an accumulation of $CO_2$ and respiratory acidosis.

D is incorrect because diabetic ketoacidosis and emphysema would lead to a mixed acidosis. (Mixed acidosis = both respiratory and metabolic: high $CO_2$ and low $HCO_3$.)

11. A patient is admitted to the medical-surgical unit for excessive diarrhea. Arterial blood gas results are pH 7.26, $PaO_2$ 97 mm Hg, $PaCO_2$ 46 mm Hg, and $HCO_3$- 15 mEq/L. Which is the first action the nurse should take in this situation?

    A. Administer Furosemide 40 mg intravenous push
    B. Infuse sodium bicarbonate 100 mEq diluted in 1 L of $D_5W$
    C. Initiate mechanical ventilation
    D. Insert an indwelling urinary catheter

    **Rationale:**

    Correct answer: B.

    This patient has metabolic acidosis due to decreased pH and decreased bicarbonate from the diarrhea, as bicarbonate ions are lost in diarrhea. The patient needs supplemental bicarbonate to restore the acid-base balance.

A is incorrect because a patient experiencing excessive diarrhea is likely dehydrated and administering a diuretic will worsen fluid loss.

C is incorrect because mechanical ventilation is used for respiratory acidosis in patients who are unable to maintain oxygen levels greater than 90%. The patient in this scenario is not experiencing a respiratory issue, and the oxygenation level is normal.

D is incorrect because insertion of a urinary catheter is not directly related to correcting the acidosis. The nurse should implement non-invasive measures when possible. Insertion of a urinary catheter increases the risk for infection.

12. Arterial blood gas results for a patient are as follows: pH 7.30, $PaO_2$ 86 mmHg, $PaCO_2$ 55 mmHg, and $HCO_3$- 22 mEq/L. What is the first intervention the nurse should implement?

   A. Assess the airway
   B. Administer bronchodilators
   C. Provide oxygen
   D. Administer mucolytics

**Rationale:**

Correct answer: A.

This patient's ABG results indicate respiratory acidosis (low pH and high $CO_2$). Assessing the airway is the nurse's greatest priority.

B is incorrect because bronchodilators may be necessary after the nurse assesses airway constriction.

C is incorrect because oxygen is not necessarily indicated unless the nurse assesses respiratory distress or hypoxia, and the $PO_2$ is normal (above 80 mmHg) in this case. The first action is airway assessment, and then oxygen can be applied.

D is incorrect because mucolytics are used if the nurse assesses thickened respiratory secretions which the patent is unable to expectorate.

13. A patient who appears nervous and is hyperventilating has the following arterial blood gas results: pH 7.49, $PaO_2$ 94 mmHg, $PaCO_2$ 31 mmHg, and $HCO_3$- 26 mEq/L. The respiratory rate is 26-26 breaths/minute. What should the nurse ask when creating the care plan?

    A. "Do you take any over-the-counter medications?"
    B. "You appear anxious. What is causing your distress?"
    C. "Do you have a history of anxiety attacks?"

D. "You are breathing fast. Is this causing you to feel light-headed?

**Rationale:**

Correct answer: B.

Anxiety and hyperventilation can lead to respiratory alkalosis, as seen in the ABG (high pH, low $CO_2$), so the nurse should help the patient identify what is causing the anxiety.

A is incorrect because assessing medications does not address the hyperventilation and anxiety and will not identify what is causing the acidosis.

C is incorrect because assessing a history of anxiety attacks will not identify what is causing the acidosis. Assessment of the here-and-now is the priority ahead of assessment of the past. The nurse should avoid asking "yes/no" questions.

D is incorrect because asking about the patient's breathing will not identify what is causing the acidosis. Asking open-ended questions will elicit more information from the patient than using "yes/no" questions.

14. A patient who was admitted for hypoparathyroidism is complaining of tingling and numbness in the fingers and

around the mouth. Which statement is most appropriate for the nurse to make?

A. "Have you been taking extra potassium supplements?"
B. "We will draw some blood to check for hypocalcemia."
C. "I will check your tendon reflexes to see if you show signs of hypermagnesemia."
D. "You may be experiencing hyponatremia."

**Rationale:**

Correct answer: B.

The parathyroid glands are responsible for maintaining adequate blood calcium levels. Hypoparathyroidism causes decreased calcium levels. Signs of hypocalcemia are numbness and tingling in the extremities and the circumoral area.

A is incorrect because hyperkalemia does not cause numbness and tingling in the extremities or around the mouth.

C is incorrect because hypermagnesemia does not cause numbness and tingling in the extremities or around the mouth. Elevated blood magnesium levels can depress the central nervous system causing hypotension, decreased deep tending reflexes, and a low respiratory rate.

D is incorrect because hyponatremia does not cause numbness and tingling in the extremities or around the mouth. Nausea, muscle cramps, twitching, and confusion can result from hyponatremia.

15. The medical-surgical nurse is caring for four patients. Which patient does the nurse identify as being at increased risk for hypernatremia?

   A. 55-year-old admitted for pneumonia experiencing diaphoresis and fever
   B. 67-year-old admitted for syndrome of inappropriate antidiuretic hormone (SIADH) and lung cancer
   C. 37-year-old admitted for vomiting and diarrhea
   D. 64-year-old admitted for congestive heart failure prescribed loop diuretics

**Rationale:**

Correct answer: A.

Diaphoresis and high fever lead to water loss through the skin, which increases serum sodium levels.

B is incorrect because SIADH causes dilutional hyponatremia.

C is incorrect because vomiting and diarrhea would cause sodium and water loss.

D is incorrect because loop diuretics would cause hypovolemic hyponatremia.

16. A patient admitted for treatment of diabetic ketoacidosis (DKA) to the medical-surgical unit now has euglycemia, normal pH, and normal serum osmolality. When assessing the patient, the patient reports leg weakness. Which intervention does the nurse implement first?

   A. Consult with physical therapy
   B. Initiate fall precautions and check serum potassium
   C. Provide uninterrupted sleep periods
   D. Encourage increased dietary intake of dairy products and leafy green vegetables

**Rationale:**

Correct answer: B.

Euglycemia is a normal blood glucose. Treatment of diabetic ketoacidosis (DKA) includes administration of IV insulin (to lower blood glucose) and IV 0.9% normal saline, which raises pH back above 7.35. This treatment moves potassium back into cells, potentially causing hypokalemia. Low potassium can cause muscle weakness, which is a patient safety issue.

A is incorrect because the potassium level needs to be checked as an immediate physical need ahead of consulting another service.

C is incorrect because rest is important, but not priority.

D is incorrect because dairy and leafy green vegetables are sources of calcium, vitamin D, iron, and potassium. Serum levels need to be checked to confirm hypokalemia before initiating dietary changes.

17. A patient with a potassium level of 5.7 mEq/L is receiving oral sodium polystyrene sulfonate. After the medication is administered, which of the following does the nurse assess first?

    A. Blood pressure
    B. Peaked T waves on ECG
    C. Bowel movements
    D. Urine output

**Rationale:**

Correct answer: C.

Normal serum potassium is 3.5-5.0 mEq/L. Treatment for hyperkalemia includes administration of sodium polystyrene sulfonate (Kayexalate), which causes an exchange of potassium for sodium in the intestines. The excess potassium is then excreted via bowel movements. The medication is not effective if the patient does not have bowel movements.

A is incorrect because blood pressure may be affected by altered potassium levels, but assessing for bowel status is more important after administering this medication.

B is incorrect because tall, peaked T waves are often seen with hyperkalemia, so this would be an expected finding in a patient with a serum potassium level of 5.7 mEq/L. The question is asking specifically about the priority assessment after giving the medication.

D is incorrect because urine output is not a priority assessment when administering sodium polystyrene sulfonate.

18. The nurse is administering an IV magnesium piggyback to a patient whose magnesium level was 1.1 mEq/L.

Which of the following would demonstrate the need to stop the magnesium infusion immediately?

A. Absence of patellar reflex

B. Loose stools

C. Premature ventricular contractions

D. Increased blood pressure

**Rationale:**

Correct answer: A.

Magnesium is a central nervous system depressant. Normal magnesium is 1.3 – 2.3 mEq/L Hypermagnesemia is characterized by depressed neuromuscular transmission and absent reflexes. If hypermagnesemia is present and the infusion is not stopped, then the patient may suffer from hypotension and decreased respiratory drive, which can become a medical emergency.

B is incorrect because loose stools are not a manifestation of hypermagnesemia.

C is incorrect because PVCs are not a manifestation of hypermagnesemia.

D is incorrect because hypermagnesemia causes hypotension.

19. A 68-year-old man admitted for heart failure has a sodium level of 115 mEq/L and is acting belligerent toward staff. When the family inquires why he is not recognizing them, what is the most appropriate statement by the nurse?

    A. "He may have dementia, and being in the hospital may have made his confusion worse."
    B. "Many older adults experience confusion while hospitalized."
    C. "His sodium level is decreased, and his confusion should improve as his levels rise."
    D. "His sodium level is elevated and his behavior is due to dehydration."

**Rationale:**

Correct answer: C.

Normal sodium is 135-145 mEq/L. This patient has hyponatremia, which causes neurological symptoms when levels are below 120 mEq/L. The patient's confusion will likely resolve once his serum sodium level is corrected.

A is incorrect because dementia is irreversible and unrelated to sodium levels.

B is incorrect because, although it may be a true statement, it is dismissive and it does not answer the family's question.

D is incorrect because the patient's sodium level is low.

20. A patient admitted for a sodium level of 118 mEq/L has received a 3% normal saline infusion at 60 mL/hr for the past 15 hours. Currently the patient reports feeling fatigue and difficulty breathing. Which intervention does the nurse perform as a priority?

    A. Decrease the infusion

    B. Draw a blood sample and send to the lab to assess the current serum sodium level

    C. Assess the patient for fluid volume overload

    D. Notify the healthcare provider immediately

**Rationale:**

Correct answer: C.

A hypertonic sodium solution is administered to increase sodium levels, which can cause fluid volume overload (FVO). The nurse must assess for signs of FVO including crackles in the lungs, peripheral edema, and increased blood pressure.

A is incorrect because decreasing the infusion is appropriate, but will not correct the problem immediately. The priority is to assess for FVO and determine next steps (such as elevating the head of the patient's bed, encouraging incentive spirometry, administering diuretics, or stopping the sodium infusion completely).

B is incorrect because, although checking sodium level is appropriate, it is not a greater priority than assessing for overload. An immediate physical assessment of the lungs is more here-and-now than sending a blood sample to the lab.

D is incorrect because the nurse must collect all relevant assessment data before notifying the healthcare provider.

21. A patient admitted with pancreatitis has received potassium supplementation for 4 days due to an initial serum potassium level of 3.1 mEq/L. This morning's potassium level was 3.3 mEq/L. Which of the following should the nurse perform before notifying the healthcare provider?

    A. Assess current serum calcium level
    B. Administer sodium chloride 3% infusion
    C. Limit dietary phosphorus intake
    D. Check magnesium level

**Rationale:**

Correct answer: D.

Decreased magnesium levels can prevent potassium ions from crossing cell membranes, which results in potassium loss in the urine. Decreased magnesium levels must be assessed and corrected before potassium replacement can be effective.

A is incorrect because assessment of calcium levels is not relevant to effectiveness of potassium supplementation.

B is incorrect because administration of a hypertonic sodium solution will not increase effectiveness of potassium supplementation.

C is incorrect because phosphorus intake is not directly related to potassium supplementation and this patient is not showing signs of hyperphosphatemia.

22. A patient who had surgery 2 days ago has experienced vomiting and complains of dizziness when she stands up to go to the bathroom. After the nurse helps the patient back to bed, it is noted that the patient's blood pressure is 66/30 and her pulse is 150. Which IV fluid does the nurse hang to correct the condition?

    A. $D_5W$ at 50 mL/hr
    B. 0.9% NS wide open
    C. $D_5$ 0.45% NS at 75 mL/hr
    D. Dextran wide-open

**Rationale:**

Correct answer: B.

This patient is experiencing hypovolemia and requires a plasma volume expansion. An isotonic fluid, such as normal saline (0.9% NS), is a safe fluid and the appropriate first choice for expanding volume.

A is incorrect because $D_5W$ becomes hypotonic after it enters the bloodstream and can further drop the blood pressure. Furthermore, a rate of 50 mL/hr is insufficient to raise a systolic pressure of 66 mmHg.

C is incorrect because $D_5$ 0.45% NS is hypotonic and will leave the intravascular space, further depleting blood volume.

D is incorrect because dextran is hypertonic and should not be initiated unless an isotonic fluid is ineffective at raising the blood pressure. Administration of a hypertonic fluid at a wide-open rate can cause overhydration and fluid volume overload.

23. A patient who has been undergoing chemotherapy is now experiencing anorexia and generalized edema. When the patient asks what edema is, which response should the nurse give?

   A. "Decreased activity has caused excess fluid to accumulate in your tissues."
   B. "The edema is a common adverse reaction from chemotherapy."

C. "Lack of nutrition causes decreased protein levels in the blood, and this causes fluid to move into your tissues from your blood vessels."

D. "Chemotherapy causes increased blood pressure, which forces fluid out into your tissues."

**Rationale:**

Correct answer: C.

Low albumin (hypoalbuminemia) occurs in response to poor nutrition, which leads to decreased oncotic pressure and generalized edema (anasarca). Low protein causes fluid to move from within the intravascular space to the interstitial space, causing edema.

A is incorrect because hypoalbuminemia is the most likely cause for the edema, even though decreased activity *can* contribute to edema.

B is an incorrect response because edema is not a common reaction to chemotherapy.

D is incorrect because chemotherapy does not increase blood pressure.

24. A patient has a recent diagnosis of syndrome of inappropriate antidiuretic hormone (SIADH) and tells the nurse he has headaches, nausea, and weight gain.

Which of the following statements are appropriate for the nurse to make?

A. "Your symptoms may be due to hypovolemia."

B. "Fluid overload from the SIADH may be causing your symptoms."

C. "Supplemental IV fluids may help treat your symptoms, which may be a result of SIADH-induced fluid loss."

D. "Do you have a family history of renal failure?"

**Rationale:**

Correct answer: B.

SIADH causes excess antidiuretic hormone release by the pituitary gland, which causes fluid retention, hypervolemic dilutional hyponatremia, and clinical manifestations of headache, weight gain, and nausea.

A is incorrect because SIADH does not cause fluid depletion.

C is incorrect because SIADH causes fluid overload, not fluid loss.

D is incorrect because a family history of renal failure is not related to symptoms of fluid volume overload from

SIADH. The nurse should avoid asking "yes/no" questions, but rather focus on the here-and-now.

25. A patient is admitted to the medical-surgical unit for a potassium level of 6.0 mEq/L. The nurse knows this finding is related to which of the following?

    A. Intermittent nasogastric suction
    B. Malabsorption syndrome
    C. Acute renal failure
    D. Laxative use

**Rationale:**

Correct answer: C.

A serum potassium level of 6.0 mEq/L indicates acute renal failure. Potassium balance is regulated in the kidneys. When kidney function is impaired, they lose the ability to adequately excrete excess potassium ions into the urine.

A is incorrect because nasogastric drainage will cause a decreased potassium level.

B is incorrect because malabsorption syndrome will cause a decreased potassium level due to a lack of dietary potassium absorption.

D is incorrect because laxative abuse causes potassium loss in the stool, leading to hypokalemia.

26. The nurse on the medical-surgical floor is caring for four patients. Which patient does the nurse identify as having the greatest risk for hypermagnesemia?

    A. Patient who chronically abuses alcohol
    B. Patient with hyperparathyroidism
    C. Patient with renal failure taking antacids at home
    D. Patient with congestive heart disease, taking furosemide daily

**Rationale:**

Correct answer: C.

Normal magnesium is 1.5-2.5 mEq/L. Antacids often contain magnesium, and patients with impaired kidney function may lose the ability to properly excrete magnesium.

A is incorrect because chronic alcoholism often causes hypomagnesemia. Symptoms include neuromuscular irritability, tremors, tetany, seizures, confusion, dysrhythmias, and depression. Other causes for hypomagnesemia include GI suction, diarrhea, and abuse of diuretics or laxatives. Nursing interventions include an increase in dietary magnesium (green leafy vegetables), seizure precautions, and safety precautions.

B is incorrect because hyperparathyroidism is often associated with hypercalcemia.

D is incorrect because this patient is at risk for hypokalemia.

27. The nurse is caring for a patient admitted yesterday who sustained second-degree burns due to a house fire. Which lab result warrants the nurse to immediately notify the healthcare provider?

   A. Hematocrit 53%
   B. Arterial pH 7.31
   C. Sodium level 133 mEq/L
   D. Potassium level 6.3 mEq/L

**Rationale:**

Correct answer: D.

Burns can cause hyperkalemia in the emergent/resuscitative stage (first 24-48 hours after the injury), which can cause a life-threatening cardiac dysrhythmia. The healthcare provider should be notified immediately of this finding.

A is incorrect because the hematocrit is elevated, but this is expected in the emergent stage after a burn injury (due to fluid loss and dehydration). The nurse should also expect to see decreased blood pressure and an increased pulse. Lactated Ringers solution and/or plasma is infused rapidly for the first 8 hours, and more slowly over the next 16 hours.

B is incorrect because the pH level is low, but acidosis is expected with burns.

C is incorrect because hyponatremia is expected with burns, and a sodium level of 133 mEq/L is not as threatening as a potassium level of 6.3 mEq/L.

28. The nurse cares for a patient with Crohn's disease and a draining fistula. Which of the following should alert the nurse to notify the healthcare provider for additional medications?

   A. White blood cell count of 8100/mm³

   B. Potassium level of 2.7 mEq/L

   C. Patient weight loss of 2 kg over the past 2 weeks

   D. Decreased appetite

**Rationale:**

Correct answer: B.

Crohn's disease is an inflammatory condition of any part of the large or small intestine, usually the ileum and ascending colon. With a fistula present, the patient is at an increased risk for hypokalemia and hypomagnesemia. Hypokalemia may cause a life-threatening cardiac dysrhythmia, so the healthcare provider should be notified immediately for additional medications. Potassium can be supplemented orally (dilute in juice to prevent GI upset) or IV (concentration no greater than 40 mEq/L).

A is incorrect because the white blood cell count is normal.

C is incorrect because a weight loss of 2 kg is concerning, but not a greater priority than intervention to prevent cardiac dysrhythmias.

D is incorrect because decreased appetite is abnormal and may require further assessment or a nutritional consult, but is not a priority over the severely low potassium.

29. A female patient admitted to the medical-surgical unit from an assisted living facility has a hematocrit of 54% and serum sodium level of 154 mEq/L. Which of the following does the nurse suspect?

A. Fluid overload

B. Anemia

C. Dehydration

D. Cholelithiasis

**Rationale:**

Correct answer: C.

Hematocrit measures the percentage of red blood cells per a fluid volume of blood. Normal hematocrit is 42-52% for a man and 35-47% for a woman. Normal serum sodium is 135-145 mEq/L. Dehydration concentrates serum and falsely elevates hematocrit and also elevates sodium levels.

A is incorrect because overhydration causes decreased hematocrit and low sodium levels.

B is incorrect because anemia causes decreased hematocrit.

D is incorrect because cholelithiasis (stones in the gallbladder) does not cause elevated hematocrit and sodium levels.

30. A patient recovering from exploratory laparotomy and removal of a large intestinal tumor has a nasogastric tube and IV fluids running by pump at 150 mL/hr. Which of the following data does the nurse report to the healthcare provider?

    A. The IV pump is at an alarming high pressure
    B. Intake is 1,800 mL, NGT output is 550 mL, and urinary catheter output is 950 mL
    C. Crackles and rales auscultated in all lung fields
    D. Absence of pedal edema and increasing level of consciousness

    **Rationale:**

    Correct answer: C.

    Crackles and rales in all fields indicates fluid overload. Appropriate nursing actions include decreasing the rate of IV fluids, elevating the head of bed, encouraging incentive spirometry and notifying the healthcare provider.

A is incorrect because a high pressure alarm on the IV pump does not warrant healthcare provider notification. The nurse is responsible for assessing the patient's IV site and addressing the alarm on the pump. The nurse can make a decision to discontinue an IV and restart a new one, or replace the IV pump if needed.

B is incorrect because the output is 300 mL less than the intake, which is expected. (Insensible fluid losses through the lungs, sweat, and stool contribute to a negative fluid balance.)

D is incorrect because these are expected findings and indicate no complication.

31. A patient's recent arterial blood gas shows a current pH of 7.32. Which of the following could be the cause of this abnormal pH level? (Select all that apply.

    A. Patient with type II diabetes who takes metformin
    B. Patient with a history of cardiac disease who takes 325 mg of aspirin daily

C. Patient who was recently defibrillated for ventricular fibrillation

D. A patient with type I diabetes admitted for hyperglycemic hyperosmolar non-ketotic syndrome (HHNKS)

E. Post-operative patient after a vagotomy and antrectomy

**Rationale:**

Correct answer: A, B, C.

Metformin can cause lactic acidosis. Aspirin is a salicylate (acidic) medication which can cause metabolic acidosis. Sodium bicarbonate is kept on hand after defibrillating a patient with ventricular fibrillation because acidosis is common.

D is incorrect because HHNKS does not cause acidosis as seen in diabetic ketoacidosis (DKA).

E is incorrect because vagotomy and antrectomy is a procedure in which the gastrin-secreting portion of the stomach is removed, and the vagus nerve is severed. Alkalosis can commonly occur after this procedure.

32. A patient with renal failure is admitted with an electrolyte imbalance. Which potential complications should the nurse assess? (Select all that apply)

A. EKG changes

B. Generalized weakness

C. Hypokalemia

D. Shallow respirations

E. Paralytic ileus

**Rationale:**

Correct answer: A, B, D, E.

Renal failure contributes to several electrolyte imbalances including hyperphosphatemia, hyperkalemia, and hypermagnesemia. The EKG should be monitored for changes, abdomen assessed for decreased motility and paralytic ileus, and generalized weakness due to hyperkalemia. Magnesium can decrease the respiratory drive.

C is incorrect because renal failure causes hyperkalemia.

33. The nurse is caring for five patients on the medical unit. Hypocalcemia is a risk for which patients? (Select all that apply)

    A. 43-year-old taking glucocorticoid medication daily

    B. 32-year-old with anorexia nervosa who recently underwent a thyroidectomy procedure

C. 51-year-old with liver failure

D. 75-year-old with chronic renal failure

E. 54-year-old admitted for hyperparathyroidism

**Rationale:**

Correct answer: A, B, D.

Calcium is needed for skeletal muscle contraction and blood clotting. Hypocalcemia is a risk for patients taking glucocorticoids, post-thyroidectomy patients, and patients with renal failure. Hypocalcemia causes the nervous system to become excitable, characterized by positive Trousseau and Chvostek signs. Seizures, confusion, paresthesia, and irritability may also be present.

C is incorrect because impaired liver function does not cause low calcium levels.

E is incorrect because hyperparathyroidism would contribute to hypercalcemia, not hypocalcemia.

34. The nurse in the clinic is providing dietary education for a man whose sodium level is 156 mEq/L. Which of the

following food recommendations does the nurse offer? (Select all that apply)

A. Bacon, lettuce, and tomato sandwich on whole wheat bread

B. Baked chicken thighs with mashed potatoes and fresh steamed peas

C. Low-fat yogurt and organic smoked turkey breast

D. Baked potato with herbs and low-sodium margarine spread

E. Tuna fish sandwich with baked potato chips

**Rationale:**

Correct answer: B, D.

This patient has hypernatremia, so a low sodium diet would be prescribed. Baked chicken, potatoes, and fresh fruits and vegetables are low in sodium. Canned and frozen items contain greater amounts of sodium than fresh produce.

A is incorrect because bacon is high in sodium.

C is incorrect because dairy products and smoked items are high in sodium.

E is incorrect because canned meats, such as tuna, salmon, and chicken are high in sodium. Baked chips may contain less fat than fried chips, but are still high in sodium.

35. The nurse in the clinic is providing dietary education for a woman whose potassium level is 3.1 mEq/L. Which of the following food recommendations does the nurse offer? (Select all that apply)

    A. Hamburger and a glass of milk
    B. Vegetable and cheese omelet, puffed rice cereal
    C. Scrambled egg whites, white toast, and strawberry jam
    D. Loaded baked potato with kidney bean chili
    E. Spinach and swiss chard salad with salmon

**Rationale:**

Correct answer: A, D, E.

This patient is experiencing hypokalemia, so an increased potassium diet would be prescribed. Hamburger, milk, baked potatoes, fish, and dark leafy greens (spinach and swiss chard) are high in potassium. Other good sources of potassium include bananas, kidney beans, sun-dried tomatoes, acorn squash, dried fruits, and avocado. Potassium deficiency can cause fatigue, depression, muscular weakness, insomnia, and cardiovascular issues.

B is incorrect because a vegetable and cheese omelet is high in sodium, not potassium. Rice cereal is also low in potassium.

C is incorrect because none of the food items are high in potassium.

36. A patient is admitted to the medical-surgical unit with a sodium level 108 mEq/L. Which interventions does the nurse implement? (Select all that apply)

    A. Encourage oral water intake up to 1500 mL daily
    B. Administer 0.45% NaCl IV
    C. Administer spironolactone
    D. Seizure precautions
    E. Assess weight and I&O daily

**Rationale:**

Correct answer: D, E.

The patient is hyponatremic at 108 mEq/L. Normal serum sodium is 135-145 mEq/L. The patient should be placed on seizure precautions and fluid restriction. Weight, intake, and output should be measured daily. Hyponatremia can cause nausea, muscle cramps, increased intracranial pressure, muscular twitching, and convulsions. Hyponatremia can be caused by a prolonged low-sodium diet, vomiting, potassium-sparing diuretics, and excessive water intake.

A is incorrect because oral water intake should be limited. The patient should be encouraged to drink sodium-rich fluids, such as beef broth or tomato juice.

B is incorrect because the safest way to correct sodium depletion is PO fluid restriction or IV administration of Lactated Ringers or 0.9% sodium chloride. If ineffective, a 3% or 5% sodium chloride drip may be used.

C is incorrect because spironolactone can worsen hyponatremia.

37. The monitor technician reports morning cardiac rhythms and lab values to the nurse. Which of the

following patients does the nurse need to assess as a priority? (Select all that apply)

A. Patient with sinus rhythm and peaked T waves

B. Patient with P-R intervals of 0.18 seconds

C. Patient admitted for suspected myocardial infarction and having frequent PVCs

D. Patient with third degree heart block and a ventricular rate of 56

E. Patient with QRS duration 0.06 seconds with occasional premature ventricular contractions (PVCs)

**Rationale:**

Correct answer: A, C, D.

Peaked T waves usually indicate hyperkalemia, and hyperkalemia can cause cardiac dysrhythmias and instability. Frequent PVCs could be due to hyperkalemia and infarcted heart muscle. Third degree heart block requires a pacemaker, atropine, dopamine, and/or epinephrine and can lead to death if not treated immediately.

B is incorrect because a normal P-R interval is 0.12-0.20 seconds.

E is incorrect because a normal QRS duration is 0.04-0.12 seconds and occasional PVCs are not concerning.

38. A patient is admitted to the medical unit for fluid overload. When assessing the patient, which assessment findings should the nurse expect? (Select all that apply)

    A. Tachycardia
    B. Distended jugular veins
    C. Warm, pink skin
    D. Hypotension
    E. Generalized weakness

**Rationale:**

Correct answer: A, B, E.

Fluid overload is manifested by increased/bounding pulse, distended jugular veins, and generalized weakness. The nurse may also find crackles in the lungs, dyspnea, confusion, peripheral edema, weight gain, and seizures.

C is incorrect because the patient experiencing fluid volume overload would have pale, cool skin.

D is incorrect because the patient would have an increase in blood pressure, not hypotension.

39. The nurse is caring for 5 patients on the medical unit. While reviewing patient charts, the nurse determines that which patients are at risk for fluid excess? (Select all that apply)

    A. Patient who has an ileostomy

    B. Patient who has congestive heart failure

    C. Patient with renal insufficiency

    D. Patient requiring sterile wound dressing changes twice daily

    E. Patient TPN infusing

**Rationale:**

Correct answer: B, C, E.

Patients at risk for fluid excess include those with congestive heart failure, altered kidney function, cirrhosis of the liver, and TPN infusions.

A is incorrect because the patient with an ileostomy is at risk for deficient fluid volume due to the large amount of fluid loss which does not reach the large intestine for reabsorption.

D is incorrect because sterile dressing changed BID does not increase the risk for fluid overload.

40. The nurse is assigned to a patient receiving IV fluids. Which of the following findings cause the nurse to suspect fluid excess? (Select all that apply)

   A. Pulmonary edema
   B. Low hematocrit
   C. Hypertension
   D. Low central venous pressure (CVP)
   E. Increased hemoglobin

**Rationale:**

Correct answer: A, B, C.

Fluid excess will cause pulmonary edema or rales, dilutional low hematocrit, and increased blood pressure or hypertension.

D is incorrect because fluid excess will cause increased CVP.

E is incorrect because fluid excess will cause decreased hemoglobin.

41. The nurse on the medical unit is caring for 5 patients. Which patients does the nurse identify as being at risk for hyperkalemia? (Select all that apply)

    A. Patient with kidney failure
    B. Patient requiring nasogastric decompression
    C. Patient with Addison's disease
    D. Patient taking spironolactone
    E. Patient with diabetic ketoacidosis

**Rationale:**

Correct answer: A, C, D.

Patients with renal failure are at risk for hyperkalemia due to the kidneys' inability to excrete potassium. Addison's disease is an adrenal disorder characterized by decreased secretion of adrenal hormones (mineralocorticoids, glucocorticoids, and androgens.) Addison's disease causes sodium, blood volume, and blood glucose to decrease and potassium to rise. Spironolactone (a potassium-sparing diuretic) can cause hyperkalemia and hyponatremia.

B is incorrect because nasogastric suction can cause hypokalemia.

E is incorrect because diabetic ketoacidosis causes hypokalemia. DKA treatment requires IV insulin, IV fluids and potassium replacement.

42. The nurse is providing dietary teaching to a patient with hypomagnesemia. The nurse instructs the patient to consume which of the following foods? (Select all that apply)

    A. Peas
    B. Oranges
    C. Cauliflower
    D. Peanut butter
    E. Canned white tuna

**Rationale:**

Correct answer: A, C, D, E.

Common food sources of magnesium include nuts, peas, cauliflower, peanut butter, canned white tuna, spinach, milk, wheat, and yogurt.

B is incorrect because oranges are high in potassium.

43. A patient is admitted to the hospital for hypokalemia. Her history reveals 4 days of vomiting and diarrhea prior to admittance. Which foods does the nurse instruct the patient to increase intake of? (Select all that apply)

    A. Applesauce
    B. Cucumber slices
    C. Orange juice
    D. Bananas
    E. Avocados

**Rationale:**

Correct answer: C, D, E.

Foods high in potassium include orange juice, bananas, avocados, beans, chickpeas, lentils, and raisins.

A is incorrect because applesauce is low in potassium.

B is incorrect because cucumber is low in potassium.

44. A patient is admitted to the emergency room with dry mucous membranes, lethargy, and restlessness. Upon assessment, the nurse finds tented skin turgor. Which of the following could the nurse suspect? (Select all that apply)

   A. Hypernatremia
   B. Dehydration
   C. Hypokalemia
   D. Hypercalcemia
   E. Hyperphosphatemia

**Rationale:**

Correct answer: A, B.

Hypernatremia and dehydration are both manifested by tented skin turgor, dry mucous membranes, lethargy, and restlessness.

C is incorrect because hypokalemia is associated with muscle weakness, paresthesia, and cardiac dysrhythmias.

D is incorrect because hypercalcemia is associated with muscle weakness, lack of coordination, and constipation.

E is incorrect because hyperphosphatemia is associated with muscle twitching and tetany.

45. The nurse is caring for a patient with hypoparathyroidism and pancreatitis. The patient is confused and irritable, and the nurse suspects hypocalcemia. Which of the following are appropriate actions the nurse can take for this patient? (Select all that apply)

   A. Assess for a sedative effect on the central nervous system
   B. Ensure adequate daily vitamin D intake
   C. Administer calcitonin
   D. Initiate seizure precautions
   E. Delegate to the nursing assistant to check Trousseau's and Chvostek's signs
   F. Observe for tetany

**Rationale:**

Correct answer: B, D, F.

Vitamin D helps regulate calcium levels by facilitating the reabsorption of calcium from bones and enhancing calcium absorption from the GI tract. Seizure precautions are indicated for hypocalcemia. Tetany is a sign of hypocalcemia.

A is incorrect because hypercalcemia would depress the CNS.

C is incorrect because calcitonin will decrease serum calcium levels.

E is incorrect because these assessments cannot be delegated to the nursing assistant.

46. The nurse is talking with a patient after reviewing significant lab results. Which of the following statements are appropriate? (Select all that apply)

    A. "Your total serum calcium 10.1 mg/dL, which falls within the normal range."

    B. "Since your magnesium level is 0.8 mEq/L, you'll need to increase your intake of green leafy vegetables and nuts and we will implement safety precautions."

    C. "Your sodium level is 128 mEq/L, which could be caused by frequent Alka-Seltzer use."

D. "Your serum potassium is 3.9 mEq/L, which is within the normal range."

E. "Your phosphorus level is 2.5 mg/dL, which is higher than normal. We will decrease dairy in your diet and reassess in a few days."

**Rationale:**

Correct answer: A, B, D.

The normal range of total calcium is 8.6-10.2 mg/dL. The normal range of magnesium is 1.3-2.3 mEq/L and green leafy vegetables and nuts are a good source of magnesium. Hypomagnesemia can cause neuromuscular irritability and confusion, so safety precautions are necessary. The normal range of potassium is 3.5-5.0 mEq/L.

C is incorrect because Alka-Seltzer is high in sodium and would not cause hyponatremia.

E is incorrect because the normal range of phosphorus is 3.0-4.5 mg/dL. A patient with hypophosphatemia would benefit from increased dairy products in the diet.

47. When caring for a patient with strict I&O ordered, which of the following does the nurse count as fluid intake? (Select all that apply)

    A. Tube feeding formula

    B. Pureed vegetables

    C. IV fluids

    D. Ice chips

    E. Jell-O

    F. Pudding

**Rationale:**

Correct answer: A, C, D, E.

Tube feeding formula, IV fluids, ice chips, and Jell-O are all considered fluid intake. Anything that is liquid at room temperature is counted as fluid intake.

B is incorrect because pureed vegetables are not liquid at room temperature, and thus are counted as solid intake.

F is incorrect because pudding is considered a solid.

48. The nursing student is learning about acid/base imbalances. Which of the following conditions does the

student learn can cause respiratory acidosis? (Select all that apply)

A. Asthma

B. Hyperventilation

C. Pulmonary emboli

D. Sedatives

E. Pneumonia

**Rationale:**

Correct answer: A, C, D, E.

Asthma, pulmonary emboli, sedatives, and pneumonia can all cause respiratory acidosis due to the trapping of $CO_2$ or inadequate gas exchange.

B is incorrect because hyperventilation causes respiratory alkalosis. (Hypoventilation can cause respiratory acidosis due to decreased $CO_2$.)

49. The nursing student is learning about acid/base imbalances. Which of the following conditions does the student learn can cause metabolic acidosis? (Select all that apply)

A. Malnutrition

B. Renal insufficiency

C. Diabetes

D. Atelectasis

E. Cushing's Syndrome

**Rationale:**

Correct answer: A, B, C.

Metabolic acidosis can be caused by malnutrition, renal insufficiency, and diabetes. Other potential causes of metabolic acidosis include salicylate toxicity, cold stress, and shock.

D is incorrect because atelectasis can cause respiratory acidosis.

E is incorrect because Cushing's Syndrome causes metabolic alkalosis. Addison's causes metabolic acidosis.

50. The nurse is caring for a patient admitted for metabolic alkalosis. The nurse knows which of the following conditions can cause metabolic alkalosis? (Select all that apply)

A. Hypovolemia

B. Diuretic use

C. Addison's disease

D. Excessive vomiting

E. Plumbism

## Rationale:

Correct answer: A, B, D.

Metabolic alkalosis can be caused by hypovolemia, diuretic use, and vomiting.

C is incorrect because Addison's causes metabolic acidosis.

E is incorrect because plumbism (lead poisoning) does not cause alkalosis. Plumbism causes irritability, sleepiness, and increased intracranial pressure.

Made in the USA
Monee, IL
22 August 2022

12154122R00075